The Truth About
Mental Illness

The Truth About Mental Illness

Two Sufferers *Finally* Speak Out

Mary and Daniel Hann

iUniverse, Inc.
New York   Bloomington   Shanghai

The Truth About Mental Illness
Two Sufferers *Finally* Speak Out

iUniverse books may be ordered through booksellers or by contacting:

iUniverse
1663 Liberty Drive
Bloomington, IN 47403
www.iuniverse.com
1-800-Authors (1-800-288-4677)

Because of the dynamic nature of the Internet, any Web addresses or links contained in this book may have changed since publication and may no longer be valid.

ISBN: 978-0-595-49984-7 (pbk)
ISBN: 978-0-595-61329-8 (ebk)

Printed in the United States of America

This book is dedicated to

Dr. Shar Edmunds

All I get is trouble all day long;
Every morning brings me pain.

-Asaph (Psalm 73:14)
New Living Translation

Contents

FOREWORD 1

One of the great privileges God has given me in my retirement from full time ministry with Queensland Baptists has been to share the pathway for a short time on the journey of mother and son, Mary and Daniel Hann. Both Mary and Daniel suffer the darkness and loneliness of depressive illness. Their sense of despair is multiplied by the simplistic advice of well-intentioned people, especially Christians, who have never been down their road.

Unless you have personally experienced depression and some of its extension disorders, you cannot understand what the sufferer goes through. We can live beside a person with the illness, observe the twists and turns of their dark journey, and we will still be ignorant of their experience of life. We can minister medically and pastorally, and see its huge variety of manifestations, a variety as wide as the personalities of the sufferers, and feel we empathise. However even then we will only be sympathising. Mental illness is a solitary confinement, a lonely experience. As much as we try to come close, we will always be as a visitor looking through bars.

As a young pastor in my first church, I had no real contact with people suffering mental illness. I held the usual cliché that mental illness was a problem of the person without Christ. Once a person became a Christian, this should be dealt with either instantaneously or certainly over time. My second church put cure to these glib and incorrect ideas. Some of the keenest believers in that church suffered depressive illnesses. The extent of the disabling varied according to the sufferer, and their families suffered as a result. Interestingly the vast majority of their children became sincere Christians. The kids could see Christ in the midst of the depression.

Although I haven't personally experienced the kind of mental illness that Mary and Daniel have, I do have some insight into how it might feel. I experienced a stress breakdown in the 1980s from overwork. I was doing work I should have left to the Lord! The feeling of powerlessness was frightening and overwhelming. However it cast me upon Christ in a way that saved and transformed my ministry. I still thank God for the residual weakness it has left.

My reading of Christian history has led me to believe that God has regularly used folk with different forms of depressive illness to a greater extent than He has used people in good mental health. I'm sure this is because such people are cast upon the Lord's strength. They know they can't do it themselves.

This book by Mary and Daniel Hann is essential reading. I urge you to read their story and experiences. Read and try to take in what they have learned from their journey. You won't be able to share their shoes. Nobody but Christ can do this. But you may gain a little more patience and understanding for the lot of the large number of people who journey through life with this debilitating affliction.

Jim Kitson
Retired Baptist Pastor

FOREWORD 2

Mental illnesses are among the least understood and, therefore, most stigmatised realms of experience. They are hard on the people who suffer them and hard on the people around them. In my work as both a medical practitioner and a psychotherapist I regularly witness the excruciating impact of mental illness on individuals and families. On the other hand my work also affords me a window into the heroic struggle that can often bring out what is best in people. It's at this level that I am constantly reminded how mysterious life is, humbled and delighted by the unpredictable strengths and capacities that can emerge in the most dire of circumstances. Like the weather on the outside, so too the weather on the inside is a force to be reckoned with.

In their writing Mary and Daniel capture the overwhelming and debilitating impact of mental illness in a style that is simple, explicit and deeply touching. With good-humoured transparency they document their difficulties and struggles. Their writing reflects their very deep Christian faith along with an equally great trust: that greater understanding of mental illness by the general public can be achieved through honest disclosure of their personal lives. This, to my mind, is an act of exquisite generosity, immense courage and ultimate humility in the service of a power greater than any of us: compassion. Living with a mental illness (whether as a sufferer or family member) requires, at the very least, that we grow in tolerance for behaviours that we don't understand. At best it can awaken deep empathetic understanding for both ourselves and others. In Mary and Daniel's writing I hear a powerful call to compassion and hope you will too.

Dr. Shar Edmunds
Psychotherapist

INTRODUCTION

WHO WE ARE AND WHY WE WROTE THIS BOOK

We are a mother and son who are both Christians and who both suffer from mental illness. This book came about after years and years of exasperation over the lack of understanding we have received from most people when we have tried to give honest answers to their questions about how we are going.

We both suffer from a combination of depression, obsessive-compulsive disorder (OCD), anxiety and, in Daniel's case, insomnia. Mary was unaware that she had these conditions until they were diagnosed in Daniel. She suffered from them throughout her life, but since so little was known about mental illnesses until recently, they went undiagnosed.

Daniel has had extensive medical treatment for almost ten years, whereas Mary only had medical treatment for six months. Daniel's treatment has consisted of regular counselling with psychiatrists, psychologists, psychotherapists, pastors and general practioners (GPs), eighteen months of cognitive behavioural therapy (CBT), and various anti-depressant medications and sleeping tablets.

Mary suffered a nervous breakdown that lasted several years. During that time she sought help from a GP who urged her to receive professional counselling, but she refused. He also prescribed anti-depressant medication, which she took reluctantly for six months before deciding it was not really working and was not for her.

From the above it is clear that we have very different opinions about how best to cope with our mental illnesses, and very different attitudes toward ongoing medical help. Daniel has chosen to make use of *all* the medical help available, while Mary has chosen the opposite. Yet we cannot honestly say that one of us is coping better than the other. *In spite of* all the medical help Daniel has received, he is no better off.

The aim of this book is to educate people about the reality of mental illness and how it affects the lives of sufferers, including Christians. The problem with our form of mental illness is that it is not readily observable, and so people have difficulty accepting that it exists. In our opinion the general community is gradually becoming more aware of mental illnesses like depression, but most Christians are sadly lagging behind. This is because Christians generally believe that if you are saved then you should always be able to be happy and overcome any problem.

The reality is that we live in a world cursed by God because of human sin. As a result, things can go wrong in *any* part of the body, including the brain. The very nature of mental illnesses such as depression or OCD is that they produce symptoms of excessive worry, anxiety, fear and other negative emotions in the sufferer. If you consider another illness, such as epilepsy, the sufferer is never told, while having an epileptic fit, to stop violently convulsing. Nor is he told to pull himself together and stop sinning. Common sense tells us that this is a symptom of the disease, not a deliberate choice of the sufferer.

In the same way it is ludicrous and extremely unhelpful to tell someone with depression to stop feeling unhappy, or someone with OCD to stop worrying. It is a symptom of the illness and is therefore *not* something that he or she can easily control. It is our aim to help people, especially Christians, to respond to sufferers with compassion and understanding, rather than dismissal and condemnation. We also want to ensure that fellow sufferers receive the right sort of help and are not treated as we have been for so long.

Mary and Daniel Hann
June 2007

CHAPTER 1

DEFINING MENTAL ILLNESS

It is important for us to clarify from the outset what we mean when we talk about mental illness. We are *not* talking about the *normal* emotions people experience on a daily basis in response to the circumstances of everyday life, such as work or relationship problems–even a rainy day! Nor are we referring to the emotions one feels when more serious crises occur. For example, it is natural to feel devastated, sad and depressed when a loved one dies. It may well be something that you never completely get over. But it is still not something that we would call mental illness.

We are referring to something that is *always* present, irrespective of what is happening in your life. It is a condition that pervades every area of daily living–work, relationships, recreation, social interaction, decision-making, household chores–just to name a few. It is an intense affliction that is crippling, over-whelming and life-long. It can turn the simplest of tasks into a highly stressful and often terrifying ordeal. This may sound over-dramatic, but the truth is that for the sufferer, this is how it feels. Having mental illness makes *every* aspect of life ten times harder than for the average person.

Many people question the existence of our type of mental illness. After all, there is no conclusive medical or scientific proof. **Our answer is our own experience.** We have both lived long enough with mental illness to know for a fact that the way we cope with everyday life is completely abnormal. It is outside the realm of normal human functioning, and is therefore beyond the comprehension of the vast majority of people.

Mental illness often affects people who are especially intelligent, conscientious and high achieving. It was a breath of fresh air for us when we read a book by Dr. Gaius Davies called *'Genius, Grief and Grace'*. For the first time, here was someone spelling out that not only is mental illness very real, but it has plagued the lives of some of the greatest and most respected Christian men and women in history. As John Stott writes in his foreword to the book: "He [Gaius Davies] tells us the truth, that some of God's heroes and heroines have been eccentric and neurotic, and have suffered repeated breakdowns." (p.10)

The book makes the important point that a person's temperament or personality does not change when he or she becomes a Christian. Neither is there any guarantee that God will heal us from all our infirmities. Again quoting from John Stott's foreword: "Grace does not render us immune to either physical or mental illness. Nor does God promise healing in every case.... Although God can and does heal.... he often leaves us to struggle with disability and to bear pain." (pp.9-10)

As we said in our introduction, our form of mental illness is not easily detected by others. This is because for the most part we choose to keep it hidden. Since the majority of people don't believe in the existence of mental illness, or at least don't understand it, we are reticent to tell them about it. We fear that if we *do* tell them, we will be disparaged and misunderstood. Most people make light of it and equate it with their own experiences of depression and anxiety, which are in no way comparable to what we suffer. Therefore their attempts to help us are uninformed and totally unhelpful.

The result is that when we are in public or in a social situation, we usually put on an act and pretend to be fine. There are two reasons for this. The first is that this is what people expect of us because outwardly we look perfectly normal. The second is that we don't want to burden people with our troubles. We would be extremely bad company if we *always* told people how we were really feeling! As you can imagine, keeping up this act is very draining.

Many Christians think that anxiety, worry, fear and unhappiness are sinful emotions that should have no place in the life of a believer. As John Stott put it in his foreword to the book mentioned above: "There is a tendency in some Christian circles to declare it inappropriate for Christians ever to fall sick. 'You have no business to suffer from depression', some say." (pp.9-10)

For this reason many Christians accuse us of trying to justify or excuse our sin by blaming it on our mental illness. This is very sad. For far too long, these types of feelings have been attributed *exclusively* to spiritual causes. If in fact they are the result of a physical abnormality, as we believe they often are, then this is the completely wrong approach. When Christians label these symptoms as being caused by a spiritual deficiency, they do untold damage to the sufferer, placing on him or her an extra burden of unnecessary guilt. Using the example from our introduction, it would be like saying to a person with epilepsy, 'Repent of your epilepsy!' Needless to say, such a remark would do no one any good.

There is a story recorded in the Gospel of John (chapter 9 verses 1-3) where Jesus came across a man blind from birth, and his disciples asked him whose sin it was that had brought about this condition. Jesus answered, 'It was neither that this man sinned, nor his parents ...' Christians today are guilty of a similar mindset when it comes to mental illness. When Christians read this passage, they immediately recognise the silliness of the disciples' question. Yet they don't realise that *their* faulty reasoning about mental illness is just as foolish.

There are two classic passages in the Gospels (Matthew 6:25-34 & Luke 12:22-31) upon which Christians base their view that believers should never worry or be anxious. These are discourses in which Jesus tells his disciples not to worry about the basic necessities of life (ie. food and clothing) because their Heavenly Father knows what they need and will provide it. To use these passages as proof that any form of worry or anxiety is sin is laughable and absurd. Jesus here addresses a very specific area of worry. To then apply this to mental illness shows a total lack of understanding of what mental illness entails.

Our worries do *not* revolve around our basic needs. We *do* trust our Heavenly Father to provide us with enough food and clothing. *Our* worries are of a completely different character. They are irrational, excessive and abnormal. They have nothing to do with the quality of our faith. To try and prescribe spiritual solutions, such as praying and reading the Bible more, or trusting God more, is futile. We can pray and pray until we are blue in the face, and yet the problem or worry is not necessarily taken away or even alleviated.

As we have said above, God does not always heal our sicknesses. He often allows us to suffer. This applies to mental illness, just as much as to any other type of illness. His purpose is for us to become more reliant on Him as we struggle with our weakness. A classic example of this is the great Apostle Paul, who was afflicted with a severe infirmity,[1] from which he begged God to heal him. But God denied his request, instead promising that His power would be perfected in Paul's weakness.

> Because of the surpassing greatness of the revelations, for this reason, to keep me from exalting myself, there was given me a thorn in the flesh, a messenger of Satan to torment me–to keep me from exalting myself! Concerning this I implored the Lord three times that it might leave me. And He has said to me, 'My grace is sufficient for you, for power is perfected in weakness.' Most gladly, therefore, I will rather boast about my weaknesses, so that the power of Christ may dwell in me.

(2 Corinthians 12:7-9)

---

1   The Bible does not specify what Paul's infirmity was. We are not implying that he had mental illness.

CHAPTER 2

LIVING WITH MENTAL ILLNESS

In this chapter we want to try to convey something of what it is like to have mental illness. But first there is something else we need to clarify. Up until now, we have spoken of mental illness without specifying the range of conditions we include under this umbrella term. We intend the term to cover depression, OCD, anxiety, panic attacks, social phobia, insomnia, bipolar disorder, schizophrenia, anorexia and bulimia. There are an endless variety of mental illnesses out there, but these are the most common ones that we know of. We are constantly amazed by the number and diversity of mental diseases that are being brought to our attention through the media.

The thing that all these illnesses have in common is that they significantly impair a person's ability to cope with life. There is a book called 'I Had A Black Dog' by Matthew Johnstone, which brilliantly captures with words and illustrations the nightmare of living with mental illness.[2] It is based and expands upon the metaphor invented by Samuel Johnson and famously used by Winston Churchill to describe his lifelong battle with depression. The author manages to tackle this very serious subject in a delightfully humorous and lighthearted manner. His words and pictures are simple but profound and give non-sufferers an excellent and very accurate insight into the agonies experienced by sufferers on a daily basis.

This 'black dog' follows the sufferer around wherever he goes. There are other metaphors that we could use–a big black cloud, or even a little devil. It

---

2   Since we completed writing this book, another 'black dog' book has been released. It is called 'Living With A Black Dog' by Matthew and Ainsley Johnstone.

attacks every source of happiness and every area of achievement. Its aim is to destroy you and make you miserable. It is stubborn, persistent, defiant, cunning and malevolent. It is ingenious at coming up with new ways to mess up your thinking and make you feel utterly wretched.

One of our all-time favourite movies is 'A Beautiful Mind', based on the book with the same title, by Sylvia Nasar. It tells the true story of the life of John Nash, an exceptionally gifted and famous mathematician, who won a Nobel Prize for his work. What makes his life so extraordinary is that he achieved all this *despite* suffering severely from schizophrenia. This is a disease that causes a person to have delusions and see things that aren't there. To the sufferer the delusions are very real, but they are just in his mind.

The movie poignantly portrays the suffering and torment of John Nash as he struggles with the disease. For many years his condition goes undiagnosed, but as his behaviour becomes increasingly bizarre and irrational, his wife finally contacts a psychiatrist who diagnoses his illness. He is admitted to a mental hospital for a course of shock treatment and prescribed medication. *He never overcomes his schizophrenia*, but through a lot of hard work and perseverance, and with the invaluable support of his wife, his friends, and his doctor, *he learns to live with it*. He still sees the imaginary people, but he makes a conscious decision to ignore them. This requires tremendous effort, discipline, determination and willpower. Sometimes the delusions still get the better of him, and he descends into madness all over again.

At first it may seem that schizophrenia is worlds apart from the mental illnesses we suffer from. But it's not. There are many more similarities than people realise and their impact upon sufferers' lives are just as debilitating. Although we don't *see* things that aren't there, we *are* plagued with obsessive, repetitive thoughts that are just as irrational and removed from reality. These lead to corresponding compulsions and behaviours that are no less bizarre than the behaviours of someone with schizophrenia.

In a very real sense, just as John Nash had to learn to distinguish between what was real and unreal in what he saw, so we too have to learn to distinguish between thoughts that are rational and irrational. And just as John Nash had to exert effort and willpower to ignore the things that were unreal, so we too have to exert effort and willpower to ignore our irrational thoughts, and resist the corresponding compulsions. Needless to say, this is a monumental struggle that consumes an enormous amount of energy and leaves us constantly feeling emotionally drained and physically exhausted.

Living with Insomnia

As we mentioned in our introduction, Daniel suffers from chronic insomnia, and has done for several years. Mary suffers from insomnia occasionally, although in recent times it has become more frequent. There are few things more demoralising than not being able to sleep night after night. As William Styron writes: "Exhaustion combined with sleeplessness is a rare torture." ('*Darkness Visible*', p.48) Most people experience insomnia on a rare and temporary basis. It is usually brought on by particularly stressful or upsetting circumstances and it usually passes once the crisis has eased. For most people sleep is not a problem; it's just something they do easily. But for a person with mental illness it is an ongoing problem that makes life unbearable.

We have often heard it said in the media that sleep deprivation has a similar effect on the body as consuming alcohol. It makes everything in your life harder to cope with. It leaves you feeling dazed, drained, irritable and out of sorts; it makes it much harder to concentrate and reduces your productivity; it depletes your energy and weakens your resistance to illness. Health professionals regard sleep to be as important to your well being as nutrition and exercise. So naturally if you are continually unable to sleep well then you will not be able to function optimally. Long term sleep deprivation is also known to increase your risk of major health problems such as cancer and heart disease.

Many people cannot understand why someone would struggle so much to sleep. They think if you are tired enough then you should be able to get to sleep in a reasonable amount of time. They don't understand that if you have a distressing thought stuck in your mind it makes it very hard to relax and drift off to sleep, no matter how tired you are. The anxious thought produces tension in your body, rendering sleep well nigh impossible, unless you are able to somehow banish it completely from your mind.

There is a perfect illustration of this in '*I Had a Black Dog*'. One of the pictures shows a man lying in bed at 3:20am with his eyes open and a big black dog sitting on top of him. On the wall are lines and lines of negative statements which are obviously meant to represent the thoughts that are going through the man's head and keeping him awake. The caption reads: "He [the black dog] liked to wake me up with very repetitive, negative thinking."

Rest assured that we are well acquainted with all the remedies commonly prescribed for insomnia such as warm milk, hot showers, exercise, chamomile tea, lavender oil, avoiding caffeine, etc. Daniel has left no stone unturned in seeking ways to alleviate his sleeplessness. If only a cure was that simple! All of these things may be effective to relieve *minor symptoms* but they are no match for a serious bout of OCD, anxiety or depression.

Daniel relies heavily on sleeping tablets to enable him to get off to sleep. We are not saying that he has trouble sleeping *every single night*–he does have the occasional reprieve, usually when he is so desperately tired that he can't help but sleep. But he does have trouble sleeping more often than not. He has good periods and bad periods. Often the good nights of sleep only come with the use of tablets. Daniel can't use tablets every night though because his body builds up a resistance and he has to increase the dosage to get the same effect. So although the tablets are very helpful they are not a complete solution to the problem.

When you have insomnia year after year, you build up a sizeable sleep deficit. You just keep on adding to it! This means that you feel more and more fatigued over time. Daniel sometimes takes afternoon naps to help him get through the day. The more fatigued you feel, the more you feel like you can't cope with anything. All of this makes life a living hell and is another cause for people to be compassionate, not derogatory.

CHAPTER 3

THE AGONY OF MENTAL ILLNESS

The agony of mental illness is difficult to describe. William Styron makes this point in his famous book on depression ('*Darkness Visible*') in which he writes that the pain is 'indescribable' (p.14). Styron compares his own experience of mental pain to "drowning or suffocation" but admits that "even these images are off the mark." (p.15) Ironically, Styron gives the most accurate and compelling description of the mental anguish of depression (and mental illness in general) that we have come across.

In many ways mental pain is worse than physical pain. As C. H. Spurgeon said in one of his sermons (from the book '*Majesty in Misery*', p.171): "Trouble of spirit is worse than pain of body … Pain of spirit is the worst of pain, sorrow of heart is the climax of griefs." An extreme example is John Bunyan, who is best known for writing the classic Christian allegory '*The Pilgrim's Progress*'. This poor man was plagued throughout his life with irrational, obsessive, negative thoughts. His inner torment is revealed in his spiritual autobiography '*Grace Abounding to the Chief of Sinners*'. The book is almost unbearable to read because Bunyan's mental agony is so intense and so obviously needless.

Bunyan's obsessional thoughts often lasted for months or years. Frequently he would overcome one worry, only for it to be replaced by another one worse than the last. He unfortunately put it down to his own wickedness of heart. If only someone had suggested to him that his obsessional thoughts were symptoms of his mental illness, not reflections of his poor spiritual state. What grief and guilt it could have spared him! Instead he was left to suffer the added torment of thinking *he* was responsible for his wretched condition.

The most devastating obsession that Bunyan wrestled with was the fear that he had committed the unpardonable sin (Mark 3:29, Luke 12:10) by thinking a blasphemous thought. This obsession consumed his mind to such an extent that we wonder how he managed to keep on living. That is what OCD is like. A minor, irrational thought pops into your head, quickly takes hold, and rapidly expands until it fills your whole mind so that you can think of nothing else. It can then take hours, days, weeks, months or years to overcome. And even when it is *seemingly* overcome, it may come back to torment you all over again.

Unlike poor John Bunyan, *we realise* that we are mentally ill. Even so, it is still very difficult to dislodge our troubling obsessional thoughts. They get stuck in our minds and go round and round like a mouse on a treadmill. In medical terms this is called 'brain-lock'. It is so frustrating because part of you knows the thought is totally irrational, but the greater part of you remains convinced that it is rational. People try very hard to persuade you otherwise, but you find it hard to believe them. When you are experiencing 'brain-lock' it is impossible to think rationally. You have to try to trust the judgement of others over your own.

Something people don't realise is that for sufferers of mental illness, feeling depressed or anxious is the normal state of affairs. It takes effort and discipline every day to try and push our negative thoughts aside and not let them completely debilitate us. It is a painful process, one that has no end. Since we are hardly ever in a good frame of mind, having to cope with the inevitable stresses of life is far worse for us than for normal people.

A good example of the daily struggle of mental illness is provided by the diaries, letters and poems of Melanie Woss, which have been published in a book called *'Alone By Myself'*. Melanie was a highly intelligent and talented teenager. Her grades at high school were mostly excellent and she had a promising future. She had a normal, supportive family and a few good friends. In spite of all this, she committed suicide. She suffered from depression. She tried to take her life multiple times before she died.

Melanie was a deep thinker. In one sense it is not a surprise that she suffered from mental illness. We do not think it is an overstatement to say that the *majority* of the great thinkers in history have been afflicted with some form of mental illness. The two almost seem to go hand in hand. Melanie's personality certainly fitted the mould. Her thoughts were very negative. She tried to be upbeat and convince everyone that she was doing fine, when she really wasn't. She had *moments* of happiness, but they were only fleeting. For mentally ill people, depression and pain is the norm, so any experiences of pleasure are treasured all the more. Melanie captures this very well in her writings.

The One Person who best understands the agony of mental suffering is Jesus.[3] The Bible says that Jesus was "a man of sorrows and acquainted with grief" (Isaiah 53:3). The source of His anguish was not so much the physical suffering of the cross, horrific as that was, but the fact that He "who knew no sin" (2 Corinthians 5:21) was about to take our sins upon Himself and bear the punishment for them in our place. This also meant that He would be forsaken by His Father, with whom He had enjoyed perfect fellowship for all eternity past. This caused Him to feel a severe depression of mind and spirit, such that He cried out: "My soul is deeply grieved, to the point of death" (Matthew 26:38).

Jesus in fact would have died then and there if God had not sent an angel to Him to strengthen Him, such was the extreme agony of His soul. He also sweat great drops of blood. C. H. Spurgeon said of Him: "He did not die in the garden, but He suffered as much as if He had died" ('*Majesty in Misery*', p.173). This is our greatest comfort, that Jesus, more than anyone else, knows what it is like to suffer extreme mental distress. As Spurgeon said: "Jesus can sympathise with you in all your sorrows, for He has suffered far more than you have ever suffered ..." (p.176). No tear that we shed goes unnoticed by God, as David wrote in Psalm 56 verse 8 (NLT): "You keep track of all my sorrows. You have collected all my tears in your bottle. You have recorded each one in your book."

---

3   Please note that we are not suggesting that Jesus suffered from mental illness. Jesus was the perfect Son of God and therefore was not afflicted with any diseases–physical or mental. We are simply making the point that the mental anguish of Jesus is very similar to the pain of mental illness. Jesus' suffering was caused by extreme circumstances, not by mental illness.

CHAPTER 4

SOME PERSONAL EXAMPLES OF MENTAL ILLNESS

Some of you may still be doubting whether we really have mental illness. The purpose of this chapter is to provide some personal examples to persuade you that we are telling the truth. We have chosen three examples for each of us out of the many that we experience. We have also included a fourth example of something we both struggle with. After reading them we are confident you will be convinced that we really are crazy!

Mary

1) Fans, buildings and trees

From her early childhood Mary has had intense fears about ceiling fans, buildings and trees collapsing. She often stays awake at night listening to ceiling fans, worrying that they might fall or that one or more of the blades might come off and cause serious injury or death. She also worries about there being too much weight in buildings, causing floors to give way and structures to collapse. Mary spends an inordinate amount of time taking belongings from upstairs and putting them in boxes downstairs in order to reduce her fears about the house falling down. When there are strong winds and storms, she also worries about trees toppling and crashing onto the house.

2) *Grocery shopping and packing*

Every week Mary goes through the tremendous ordeal of grocery shopping. It starts with writing the shopping list and ends with putting it all away. The whole experience fills her with dread. From the day before it makes her feel sick, depressed and weak at the knees. She is overwhelmed by the difficulty of locating and deciding on the products she wants from the ever increasing range on supermarket shelves. She gets terribly flustered and wastes a lot of time trying to find what she's looking for.

Similarly Mary struggles with packing to go away anywhere. Again she is overwhelmed by all the decisions she has to make. She is obsessive about colour coordinating her clothes and accessories. Lately, in desperation, she has limited herself to one colour to try and make the task easier. She is also obsessive about cleaning and wants the house to be clean and tidy before she leaves. In recent years she has made the family leave up to two days late for holidays. So she now gives herself two weeks to clean and pack before going away. The whole process is thoroughly debilitating.

3) *Approval addiction and unassertiveness*

Mary suffers acutely from approval addiction and unassertiveness—two conditions which go hand in hand. When you suffer from approval addiction, being assertive is virtually impossible. You fear that by saying no to someone you will disappoint them and lose their good opinion. It's not that Mary craves popularity, it's just that she is overly conscientious about wanting to do the right thing by everyone. This fear is not entirely unfounded–controlling people often *do* respond in a hostile and ungracious manner. The result is that Mary ends up doing a lot of things she doesn't want to do and is not cut out to do. She also has a lot of her time wasted by people who take advantage of her unassertiveness. She finds it terribly hard to tell people that she has things to do and can't spare a lot of time. And on the rare occasions when she *does* summon the courage to tell them, she doesn't do it assertively enough and they don't take any notice. Mary gets tied up in knots in social situations, worrying excessively about what is the right thing to do and what people think of her.

Daniel

1) Germs

When Daniel was first diagnosed with OCD, he was suffering from the classic symptom of the fear of germs. He worried excessively about passing on germs and making other people sick or even causing their deaths. As a result he would wash his hands frequently and engage in other rituals to try and avoid contamination.

One outstanding example of this is Daniel's 'chair phobia'. When Daniel would go to the toilet, he feared that if any of his clothes touched the surface of the toilet, they would become contaminated. To reduce the risk of spreading the germs, Daniel got into the habit of sitting in one particular chair after going to the toilet. Over time he became convinced that that chair was crawling with germs! As a result he feared other people sitting in that chair. He also feared that if he sat in that chair and then went to somewhere like church, where there were elderly people, they would get sick and die! Daniel was seeing a psychologist at the time, and as part of the cognitive behavioural therapy (CBT) program, she made Daniel sit in the chair and then go and sit in our elderly next door neighbour's house! This is a key aspect of CBT–confronting one's fears and seeing that you don't get the result you were dreading. It will come as no surprise to you that our next door neighbour is still alive and kicking!

Another way Daniel tried to deal with his 'toilet phobia' was to have a specific set of clothes for going to the toilet. This meant that before going to the toilet he would change out of the clothes he was wearing into his 'toilet clothes'. Afterwards he would change back into the clothes he was previously wearing. He kept his toilet clothes on a specific chair in his room, and so naturally he assumed that that chair was contaminated too. As you can imagine he was not fond of using public toilets! He also felt the need to wash his clothes more often than was necessary, so he generated an enormous amount of laundry, much to his mother's annoyance!

Thankfully, over a number of years, Daniel got his obsession with germs under control, to the point that it now rarely troubles him. But other obsessions were only too happy to take its place! Sadly, his success rate with these has not been as high.

2) Doubts about the Bible

For many years Daniel struggled relentlessly with doubts about the historical authenticity of the Bible, especially the gospels. He was afraid that the gospel narratives might only be fictional. As you can imagine, for a Christian, this was a particularly profound torment. It took Daniel about five years to gain some victory over this fear, only for it to be replaced by another one which was just as severe. This second wave of doubts concerned the accuracy of the Biblical text that we have today. He feared that there might be errors in it due to the fact that the original manuscripts have been copied over and over again through the centuries. Daniel became obsessed with buying expensive books on these subjects to try and allay his fears. On the positive side, Daniel is now an expert on the historical reliability of the gospels and textual criticism!

3) Soccer and weights

Daniel has always been very conscientious about his spiritual life, to the point of being obsessive. There are two standout examples of this. The first concerns his love of soccer. Daniel regularly attends local soccer matches with his father. Several years ago his team was not faring so well, especially in their home matches. Over time Daniel became convinced that the team was losing because of him! It seemed that whenever he went to watch them, they would lose, and whenever he didn't go, they would win (or at least draw). Daniel thought that he cared too much about the result and had made soccer an idol. He thought that God was confirming this by causing his team to lose each time he went. One time Daniel was even brought to tears after his team had lost yet again because he thought that he was responsible! The compulsion for Daniel was to stop attending the games, and he did this at least a few times. But you will be happy to know that with the encouragement of his psychologist, as well as his family and friends, he persisted in going, and gradually the pattern turned around, and he saw that he wasn't the cause after all!

The second example concerns Daniel's decision to take up a gym membership. He has always been very skinny and wanted to build up his physique. He had just finished his university studies and had a long summer holiday ahead of him, so it seemed like a good opportunity to do it. But, from the moment Daniel signed up, he was swamped with guilt about it. Again he feared that it would become an idol–that he would spend too much time at the gym and become obsessed about his body. He persisted in going to the gym for three weeks. During that time he sought counsel from his family and from trusted Christian friends, all of whom unanimously said that they thought it was a fine thing for him to do. There was no hint of disapproval from anyone. But he was still not convinced–he continued to obsess about it night and day. And so, at the end of those three weeks, to the dismay of everyone, he cancelled his membership. A short time later he began doing weights at home but even this caused him undue guilt. This issue still troubles him today.

A combined example–singing and soccer

We both suffer from extreme performance anxiety–Mary in relation to singing in church and Daniel in relation to playing competitive soccer. We are not talking about the *normal* nerves that people get before they have to perform in some way. Our anxiety goes way beyond that. For us it is crippling, affecting our performance and robbing us of any enjoyment of the activity. We both doubt our abilities unnecessarily and end up fulfilling our fears about not performing to a certain standard. Needless to say this is a constant source of frustration. Even when it's over it's not really over because we then analyse our performance in minute detail, tormenting ourselves by dwelling on our mistakes. As you can imagine, this is a terribly painful process.

When Daniel first started playing soccer at the age of eleven, he didn't have any problem with nerves. He played so well that year that he won the award for the 'Best and Fairest' player in the team. Yet, almost overnight, from one year to the next, his confidence deserted him and he has struggled ever since. When Daniel was in Year 12 he had aspirations of being a professional player, so he joined a serious club. For that whole season Daniel got so nervous before each game that he couldn't sleep the night before. As a result he didn't play anywhere near his capability. This disappointment was a major part of his very severe depression that year. He subsequently resigned himself to the fact that he did not have the mental strength to pursue a professional career. It is sad but true that Daniel's popularity in each team fluctuated according to how well he played.

For both of us, singing and soccer respectively are major passions in our lives. They are the activities in which we most desire to excel. We both continually contemplate giving up and at times we have. But sooner or later we return to it and give it another go. We never truly give up.

Summary

These examples illustrate two important points. The first is that with certain OCD symptoms (such as Mary's ceiling fan phobia or Daniel's germ phobia) the major worry is about *other* people coming to harm, more so than yourself. The second is that OCD attacks those things that are most important to you (such as wanting to do the right thing by people or religious beliefs)—the things that are foundational to your happiness. This exemplifies the cruel nature of mental illness.

If any of you still had doubts about the reality of mental illness, the examples we have given above should be conclusive. As we wrote about them it brought home to us just how absurd (and sometimes comical) our worries are. Yet they are nevertheless very real and very painful. If these stories from our own experience have not convinced you, then we are afraid that nothing ever will.

CHAPTER 5

WORK AND MENTAL ILLNESS

Mentally ill people feel the curse of work much more than the average person. In the beginning, work was part of God's perfect creation. God designed us to work and to find fulfilment in it. But after Adam and Eve sinned, God cursed the ground, making work more difficult and less enjoyable from then on. As God said in Genesis 3:17-19: "Cursed is the ground because of you. In toil you will eat of it all the days of your life. Both thorns and thistles it shall grow for you … By the sweat of your face you will eat bread till you return to the ground …"

Most people take work in their stride. It is something that they can cope with and manage quite happily. We are not saying that work is *never* stressful or unpleasant for them, but on the whole, it doesn't cause them undue anxiety or depression. This is not the case for people with mental illness. They are either unable to work at all or their capacity to work is severely limited.

Before Mary got married, she worked full time as a secretary. She found it very difficult to cope with. She knew there was something wrong with her, but she didn't know what it was. Any attempts to confide in people about how she was feeling were met with derision, so she kept quiet and struggled along as best she could. After she married, she was able to be just a wife and mother, but she felt guilty about not contributing to the family finances. So after a while she did take on some extra work. She continued to work at least part time up until recently when, with the full support of her family, she decided it wasn't worth the stress it was causing her.

Daniel went to university for six years and completed two bachelor degrees in Commerce and Law. His intention was to go into full time work as an accountant at the end of his course. During one semester he took on some part time work at H&R Block as a tax consultant. This was Daniel's first experience of work and it was a nightmare. The pressure and stress were unbearable. As a result of this experience it gradually dawned on Daniel that he would not be able to cope with the demands of being a full time accountant. At that time he successfully applied for a disability support pension. He now works part time as a delivery driver and printing assistant.

When you are mentally ill, it is terribly hard to cope with the pressures of work. Because mental illness is usually so difficult to detect, people expect you to do your job with the same level of competence as a person with a normal, healthy mind. This is unrealistic and unfair. It's like expecting someone with a broken arm to log trees as easily as someone with two good arms. It's an extremely tough ask!

Often people with mental illness are misjudged as being lazy because they either don't work at all or only work part time. This is entirely unjustified. For mentally ill people, *any* work they do is an achievement and they should be commended for it, however little it is, not looked down upon for not doing more. To work at all with such a debilitating illness and under such duress is a very valiant thing to do. For Daniel, every day of work he gets through without any major mishaps is a miracle.

Far from being lazy, most people with mental illness are extremely hard working and conscientious. They are perfectionists in everything they do. If they have a task that they feel confident with, they will do it to the best of their ability, even to the point of putting in extra hours for no pay. It is a different story if they have a task that they don't know how to do, or don't feel confident with. Then they would rather not do the task at all, than do it to a standard that they consider to be not high enough. People with mental illness feel the disappointment and humiliation of making mistakes more keenly than most. They really take it to heart. Therefore they will do their utmost to avoid being put in situations where they are out of their depth and likely to make a fool of themselves.

Speaking of making mistakes, this is one of the biggest fears for mentally ill people at work. They worry excessively about mistakes they may or may not have made and what the consequences will be. The things they worry about are usually very minor but their diseased minds turn them into something major. The worries often play on their minds for the rest of the day and evening and make it impossible to get a good night's sleep. This impacts on how they feel and cope the next day. This pattern is repeated day after day. It is a vicious cycle.

One extreme example of this occurred during Daniel's time at H&R Block. While working on a Saturday afternoon he tripped over a power cord, unplugging it and causing his computer to shut down. He switched it back on and checked his work to see if any information had been lost. It hadn't. He finished his work and went home. As the evening progressed he began to worry that maybe the loss of power *had* affected his work. By the next morning he had made himself ill with worry, to the point that he couldn't face going to church. He stayed in bed until his parents left for church, then he got up, got dressed and drove into work. He spent a couple of hours re-entering data to ease his fear that some information might have been lost. The whole time Daniel knew that what he was doing was totally irrational and needless. But at the same time the obsession was so strong that he felt compelled to do it.

People with mental illness suffer from a general lack of confidence. As a result, even doing simple tasks can cause them high levels of anxiety. This in turn impairs their ability to think clearly and to make sound judgements. Their common sense deserts them and they flounder and panic. Consequently they can't do the job as competently as a normal person. This has nothing to do with a lack of intelligence. It's the anxiety that prevents them from performing to the best of their ability. We can understand how this whole process must be incomprehensible to their co-workers.

Another aspect of mental illness that makes work extra hard is having to try to put aside the negative thoughts going round and round your head in order to focus on your work responsibilities. Such thoughts are very distracting and absorb an awful lot of energy. They are also distressing and depressing. No matter how hard you try, they are nearly always present in your mind to some extent. The constant exercise of trying to silence these thoughts and concentrate on the tasks at hand makes work all the more tiring.

Mary would dearly love to be working and earning some extra income, but she feels too constrained by her lack of confidence in her abilities. Also, she already struggles enough to cope with her existing daily tasks, without having to fit in work as well. Daniel's current job was supposed to be free of stress, but this has turned out not to be the case. He finds the printing duties very stressful. When he drives, he struggles with boredom from not being able to actively exercise his mind. He is also frustrated that he is in a low-paid job where he doesn't use his tertiary qualifications.

CHAPTER 6

Responding to Mental Illness

There is a right way and a wrong way to respond to people with mental illness. Unfortunately, most people respond in the wrong way. As soon as we try to share with them something about our condition, they immediately go into fix-it mode, offering unsolicited advice and solutions, thinking that if we would only listen to them and do what they say, we would be cured. They treat us as if we are poor, dumb creatures who cannot think for ourselves and who need them to sort us out.

This kind of reaction invariably comes from people who *don't* have mental illness. Therefore they are speaking about something they don't understand. Mental illness is far too complex to be solved by such simple solutions as exercising regularly, eating healthily, praying, reading the Bible or getting a daily dose of sunshine. We already do all of these things in abundance. There is a song called *'Jerry, Stand Up'* by the band Something For Kate in which the singer offers simple but useless advice to someone who is depressed. He sings: "All you need is fresh air, a nice new suit, a walk in the park every day or two ..." If only it was that simple!

In the Bible there is a book which tells the story of a very righteous and rich man called Job, who in one day lost all of his ten children and all of his wealth. Soon after this he was afflicted with terrible sores from head to toe. Job had three friends who tried their utmost to convince him that the horrendous calamities that had come upon him were God's punishment on him for great sins he had committed. But Job maintained he was innocent of any serious wrongdoing against God. What Job's three friends were unaware of was the transaction that had taken place between God and Satan in the throne room of heaven. There God had granted Satan permission to bring calamities upon Job to test his faith.

The way Job's three friends reacted to his misery provides a good analogy for the *wrong* way most people respond to sufferers of mental illness.[4] They try to offer advice and solutions, thinking that they know all the facts when they don't. Like Job's friends, they sincerely believe they are giving the right advice, but because they don't know the *real cause* of the person's affliction, their advice is completely wrong. They don't realise that they are being judgemental, self-righteous, condescending know-alls. As Job said to one of his friends, "What counsel you have given to one without wisdom! What helpful insight you have abundantly provided!" (Job 26:3) At the end of the book God vindicated Job and rebuked his friends. God only forgave them after Job prayed for them. In the same way God will rebuke those who have responded wrongly to victims of mental illness.

There is a song by Christian artist Michael Card called '*I Will Not Walk Away*' which has a verse that aptly describes both the wrong and the right way to respond to human suffering. He sings: "Don't read me pointless poems friend, Don't diagnose, don't condescend … I need someone to weep with me." Also there is a verse in the Bible that expresses the folly of trying to jolly someone out of their depressed state: "Singing to a person who is depressed is like taking off a person's clothes on a cold day, or like rubbing salt in a wound" (Proverbs 25:20 GNB).

Ironically, a perfect example of the *right* way to respond to people suffering from mental illness is again found in the book of Job. When Job's three friends *first* heard about his personal disasters, their reaction was spot on:

> Now when Job's three friends heard of all this adversity that had come upon him, they came each one from his own place…. and they made an appointment together to come to sympathise with him and comfort him. When they lifted up their eyes at a distance and did not recognise him, they raised their voices and wept. And each of them tore his robe and they threw dust over their heads toward the sky. Then they sat down on the ground with him for seven days and seven

---

4   Again, we are not suggesting that Job suffered from mental illness. Job's misery, like Jesus', was brought on by a devastating set of circumstances.

nights with no one speaking a word to him, for they saw that his pain was very great. (Job 2:11-13)

We can testify that the people who have been the most help to us in our afflictions have been those who really listen, empathise and feel our pain. As Henri Nouwen beautifully writes:

When we honestly ask ourselves which person in our lives means the most to us, we often find that it is those who, instead of giving advice, solutions, or cures, have chosen rather to share our pain and touch our wounds with a warm and tender hand. The friend who can be silent with us in a moment of despair or confusion, who can stay with us in an hour of grief and bereavement, who can tolerate not knowing, not curing, not healing and face with us the reality of our powerlessness, that is a friend who cares. (Quoted in a book called *'The Art of Tea and Friendship'* by Sandy Lynam Clough, p.8)

Ideally, this should be the *normal* response from Christians. Jesus commanded that *love* should be the defining characteristic of the Christian church (John 13:34-35). The Apostle Paul wrote to the Galatians: "Carry each other's burdens, and in this way you will fulfil the law of Christ." (Galatians 6:2 NIV) He also wrote to the Corinthians: "And if one member suffers, all the members suffer with it." (1 Corinthians 12:26) But in our experience, tragically, this has rarely been the case. To Christians' shame, non-Christians often respond with greater love and compassion. This should not be!!

When Christians fail to acknowledge that our mental illnesses are genuine, there is a fundamental breakdown in our relationship with them. It is among Christians that we should feel *most* comfortable to share openly and honestly about ourselves. But if we know we are not going to be believed, and that we will be looked down upon, we naturally hold back. As a result we are unable to expose our *true* selves and we cannot experience the fullness of Christian fellowship that God intends. Ultimately we know that Jesus understands and loves us better than anyone on earth can. "For we do not have a high priest who cannot sympathise with our weaknesses ..." (Hebrews 4:15). What a comfort this is to our wounded souls.

CHAPTER 7

THE DEADLY SIDE OF
MENTAL ILLNESS

'I see no end to my misery but the grave.'[5]

It is a tragic fact that mental illness often ends in suicide. This is another reason why people should not downplay or dismiss the suffering of a mentally ill person. Unfortunately, suicide is a taboo topic in Christian circles. Rarely is it ever mentioned, and if it is, it is only to illustrate what they view as the ultimate outcome of someone living their life without God.

In our opinion most suicides are the result of mental illness in its severest form. As Lewis Wolpert writes in his book *'Malignant Sadness'*: "… suicidal people usually have a serious psychiatric disorder, most often depression." (p. 70) Archibald D. Hart says much the same thing in his book *'Unmasking Male Depression'*: "Suicide is largely a depression problem … You don't kill yourself just because you're bored!" (p. 4)

Obviously we do not advocate suicide. As Christians we believe that God made each one of us. He owns us and therefore only *He* has the right to terminate our lives. So clearly the act of suicide is a sin. The same principle applies to euthanasia and abortion.

While we affirm that suicide is a sin, we do not think it is in the same category as murder. It is one thing to take your own life, but it is another thing altogether to take the life of another. Because of our own experiences of the agony of mental illness, we can feel compassion for those who commit sui-

---

5   *'The Sorrows of Young Werther'*, Johann Wolfgang Von Goethe, p.69.

cide. We cannot, however, sympathise with those who kill others before killing themselves.

Kathryn Greene-McCreight in her book *'Darkness is My Only Companion'* expresses a similar sentiment. She is a Christian who suffers from bipolar disorder (or manic depression). Prior to the onset of her disease she held a very negative attitude towards suicide. As she writes: "I used to think suicide was the most selfish act anyone could perform ..." (p.45) But her attitude changed dramatically once she experienced the torment of mental illness for herself. She writes: "Now I see the matter differently, having been suicidal myself. I now think that suicide is the most pitiful act. I am no longer angry with my friends who took their lives; I feel nothing now for them except compassion, pity, and sorrow." (p.45)

Many people do regard suicide as an extremely selfish act, due to the devastation that it brings upon family and friends. While we agree with this to some extent, we think that those who hold this view fail to consider just how much pain a person must be in to even contemplate suicide. No one commits suicide lightly; rather, as Kathryn Greene-McCreight writes: "... it is a choice born of tremendously unbearable pain." (p.47) That pain is aptly summarised by a verse in the Bible: "All I get is trouble all day long. Every morning brings me pain." (Psalm 73:14 NLT)

When someone is in a suicidal state, the depth of his despair outweighs any thought of the grief he might inflict on his loved ones. He becomes convinced that his friends and family will be better off without him. This is how Kay Redfield Jamison reasoned when she was suicidal. As she writes in her book *'An Unquiet Mind'*: "I thought that ... I was doing the only fair thing for the people I cared about; it was also the only sensible thing to do for myself." (p.115)

Regrettably, most Christians regard someone who commits suicide with contempt. They automatically assume that the person must have been a great sinner. We disagree. The truth is that we are all great sinners. As the Bible says: "for all have sinned and fall short of the glory of God" (Romans 3:23). There is a story recorded in the Gospel of Luke in which Jesus was told about some people who had met with a gruesome death (Luke 13:1). Jesus responded in the following way:

"Do you suppose that these Galileans were greater sinners than all other Galileans because they suffered this fate? I tell you no, but unless you repent, you will all likewise perish. Or do you suppose that those eighteen on whom the tower in Siloam fell and killed them were worse culprits than all the men who live in Jerusalem? I tell you, no, but unless you repent, you will all likewise perish." (Luke 13:2-5)

The point is that no matter how we die, we are all sinners who need to repent. Since most suicides are primarily caused by mental illness, it is wrong to judge those who commit suicide as being more sinful than the average person. William Styron once wrote a letter to a newspaper in defence of those who commit suicide because of mental illness. He argued that suicide should not be viewed any more harshly than death from any other disease. He describes the letter in his book *'Darkness Visible'*:

"The argument I put forth was fairly straightforward: the pain of severe depression is quite unimaginable to those who have not suffered it, and it kills in many instances because its anguish can no longer be borne … but to the tragic legion who are compelled to destroy themselves there should be no more reproof attached than to the victims of terminal cancer." (p.32)

The question remains as to whether a true Christian could commit suicide, and if so, would he still go to heaven? Or would he go to hell? Is suicide an unforgivable sin? The weight of Christian opinion seems to favour the view that suicide is unforgivable and therefore condemns one to hell. For instance the famous Christian writer G. K. Chesterton once wrote: "Not only is suicide a sin, it is the sin. It is the ultimate and absolute evil …" Kathryn Greene-McCreight quotes this passage in her book (p.44) and then makes the following comment: "Chesterton's is a typical Christian view of suicide as a grave sin, even the gravest of sins." (p.45) Further on in her book she makes the observation that the Christian view of suicide is that "… it is considered to be unforgivable by God, so great is the offence." (p.47) In another passage written by Chesterton in his book called *'Orthodoxy'*, he contrasts martyrdom and suicide, and concludes by saying that they are "at opposite ends of heaven and hell." (p.55)

In our view, the 'typical Christian view of suicide' is wrong. We believe it *is* possible that a true Christian could take his own life and still go to heaven. To say that suicide is unforgivable is untenable; there is no Biblical basis for it.

There is only one sin that the Bible says is unforgivable: blasphemy against the Holy Spirit (Mark 3:29 & Luke 12:10). This clearly does not refer to suicide.

If suicide *was* unforgivable, then this would mean a Christian could lose his salvation. But this would undermine the finished work of Jesus on the cross. The Bible teaches that Jesus died once for *all* our sins–past, present and future (1 Peter 3:18). So an act of suicide by a true Christian cannot undo what Jesus has already accomplished. If a true Christian happened to be angry with some-one when he died, no one would claim that this sin would bar him from heaven. So it is inconsistent to insist that suicide is any different.

It is terrible but true that if an unsaved person commits suicide, he *will* go to hell. Not because suicide is the worst of sins, but simply because *all* unsaved people go to hell when they die. We know this will offend many people, but it is what the Bible teaches. John 3:36 (NIV) says: "Whoever believes in the Son has eternal life, but whoever rejects the Son will not see life, for God's wrath remains on him." So when an unsaved person with mental illness commits sui-cide, thinking it is the only way to end his pain, he unknowingly brings upon himself a fate that is far worse than he could ever have imagined. **This** is the biggest tragedy of suicide.

RECOMMENDED READING AND BIBLIOGRAPHY

If you would like to read more about mental illness we highly recommend all of the following books, most of which have been referred to throughout this book:

Bunyan, John. *Grace Abounding to the Chief of Sinners*. Great Britain: Penguin Classics, 1987.

Carlson, Dwight L, MD. *Why Do Christians Shoot Their Wounded? Helping (Not Hurting) Those with Emotional Difficulties*. USA: InterVarsity Press, 1994.

[The above book has a remarkably similar message to our own. We want to make it clear that we did not come across this book until *after* we had finished writing our own. It gives the same message, but in greater detail, and with more medical information, as the author is a psychiatrist.]

Davies, Dr. Gaius. *Genius, Grief and Grace: A Doctor looks at Suffering and Success*. Scotland: Christian Focus Publications, 2003.

Deveson, Anne. *Tell Me I'm Here*. Australia: Penguin Books, 1998.

Greene-McCreight, Kathryn. *Darkness Is My Only Companion: A Christian Response to Mental Illness*. USA: Brazos Press, 2006.

Hart, Archibald D. *Unmasking Male Depression*. USA: W Publishing Group, 2001.

Jamison, Kay Redfield. *An Unquiet Mind: A Memoir of Moods and Madness*. Great Britain: Picador, 1995.

Johnstone, Matthew. *I Had a Black Dog.* Sydney: Pan Macmillan Australia, 2005.

Johnstone, Matthew and Ainsley. *Living With A Black Dog.* Sydney: Pan Macmillan Australia, 2008.

Nasar, Sylvia. *A Beautiful Mind.* Victoria: Faber and Faber, 1999.

Styron, William. *Darkness Visible.* London: Vintage, 2004.

Wigney, Eyers & Parker (ed). *Journeys With The Black Dog: Inspirational stories of bringing depression to heel.* Australia: Allen & Unwin, 2007.

Wolpert, Lewis. *Malignant Sadness: The Anatomy of Depression.* London: Faber and Faber, 2006.

Woss, Melanie. *Alone By Myself: The moving diary of a teenager who lost the battle with depression.* Victoria: Penguin Books, 2002.

The following books were also quoted from but are not specifically about mental illness:

Chesterton, G. K. *Orthodoxy.* USA: Relevant Books, 2006.

Clough, Sandy Lynam. *The Art of Tea and Friendship.* Oregon: Harvest House Publishers, 2003.

Goethe, Johann Wolfgang Von. *The Sorrows of Young Werther.* England: Penguin Books, 1989.

Spurgeon, C. H. *Majesty in Misery Vol.1 Dark Gethsemane.* Edinburgh: The Banner of Truth Trust, 2005.

Songs we quoted from:

Card, Michael. 'I Will Not Walk Away,' *The Hidden Face of God.* Grand Rapids, MI: Discovery House Music, 2006.

Something For Kate. 'Jerry, Stand Up,' *The Murmur Years: The Best of Something For Kate.* Australia: Sony BMG Music Entertainment, 2007.

Movies discussed:

A Beautiful Mind. Universal Studios and DreamWorks LLC, 2001.

www.ingramcontent.com/pod-product-compliance
Lightning Source LLC
Chambersburg PA
CBHW050345290526
45785CB00006B/2637